poetry

Dennis Rivard

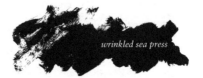

wrinkled sea press

sidelong glances

wrinkled sea press
P.O. Box 234
S. Orleans, Massachusetts 02662
info@wrinkledsea.com

ISBN: 978-1-7377477-0-3

Editor: Gerry Grenier
Associate Editor: Paul Cordeiro

Cover photo by Amy Whittenburg
Book design by Charita Patamikakorn

Publisher's Note

Dennis Rivard has been practicing the fine art of poetry for more than 50 years. Given the quantity and quality of his work, it is surprising that he has been published only in limited-distribution publications. Now, as he grapples with a diagnosis of early Alzheimers, *Sidelong Glances* is his long overdue debut to a wider audience.

This volume features a selection of Dennis's past and recent work. In its words and rhythms, we are struck by Dennis's poignant observations on this maze of seeming-wonders that surrounds us—as well as the pain and confusion caused by his memory loss.

How this book came to be is a story in itself. In 1971 I was a nerdy high school senior in the Massachusetts port city of New Bedford. When the class yearbook, the *Crimson Log*, came out in May of that year, I flipped through and found a poem that captivated me—and that poem stayed with me for decades.

The poem was "My Christmas" by Dennis Rivard (he was a fellow senior, but I didn't really know him; he ran with the "cool" crowd). "My Christmas" described a dystopian view of the holiday, inspired by novelist George Orwell's

1984. Nearly every Christmas season I pulled out my yearbook and, while reliving my high school memories, read Dennis's poem again and again. I shared the poem with co-workers, I stuck it up on the refrigerator.

As the years went by, I wondered what became of Dennis. How did his life turn out? Was he a famous poet? Did he abandon his passion and become a high-flying CEO? It was nearly half a century before I learned the answer. Prompted by a call to sign up for the New Bedford High School Class of 1971 reunion in March 2020, I googled Dennis, and his parents' obituaries led me to what I hoped was still a current address in White River Junction, Vermont. I decided to write a very belated fan letter. The response was a stack of poems, some handwritten, some typed, and a letter. Dennis explained that he had never stopped writing, and, in fact, had penned nearly 700 poems.

We began a phone and letter correspondence during the summer of 2020. Undaunted by his diagnosis, he was still producing poetry, and lots of it. Then I got an idea. I'd been in publishing all my life (life sciences and engineering), was about to retire, and felt the need to do something that mattered. Driven by the power of Dennis's work, I had a late-night inspiration (aided by two Bombay Sapphire martinis!) to publish his poetry. "Wrinkled Sea Press," a labor of love, was born.

Sidelong Glances is not only Dennis's debut, but Wrinkled Sea's as well. The circle is now complete. I extend my deepest gratitude to Associate Editor Paul Cordeiro (haiku poet extraordinaire) for serving as Dennis's unofficial archivist and as my guiding light as we culled through the collection. Thanks also to Dennis's sister, Diane Rivard McCarthy, for her insights into Dennis's early life and her unwavering support.

And, of course, my deepest gratitude to Dennis for responding to that initial letter and for bearing with me during this fulfilling journey. More to come.

Gerry Grenier
Wrinkled Sea Press
Orleans, Massachusetts
September 2021

Author's Note

My heartfelt thanks go out to the extraordinary people
who worked so diligently on this labor of love. Gerry,
Paul, Diane. All good and loyal friends. Years of scattered
appearances in a variety of small poetry mags and
journals. Now this modest but heartfelt book.

Dennis Rivard
Windsor, Vermont
September 2021

Poems

Brain Cells

Some of my brain cells,

they've clumped, I think,

into some unofficial

faction. They've split off

into some secret

club I'm not part of.

And it's clear they

don't want me

visiting. Let alone

joining. Shady faction

indeed. And

I don't even know

where they hold

their meetings.

Close To The Surface

River frozen on the right
hand side, but running
along the left side
nicely. Probably something
to do with the shade
and sunshine. Sometimes logic
is deep down below
the surface, well-prepared
to remain unseen.
A fish understands.
Other times, it's so close to
the surface—in clear sight—
that it's catchable
with just your two bare hands.

It was just a little fly-speck
of a town, called Earth. Not everyone
even knew it existed. Some maps
didn't even feature it. Classification:
Insignificant. Its only claim to fame:
how the dominant species killed
so many of each other.
"Highly evolved," is how they saw
themselves. So said the great
investigation squads. Killed their own
kind by the hundreds
of thousands. We know this. We're
just not sure why. In telescopes,
they looked like tiny
pests. And yes, you're right—
their arrogant delusions
made them somewhat
significant after all. In fact, the final
great explosion was looked
upon as something fairly
tragic. Seen as a notable shame
in certain far-flung corners of our
disapproving universe.

No Fear, Of Flying

At times I'm flying
by instruments.
Sometimes I'll be talking
on the radio to
somebody in the control
tower. Sometimes
I'm just floating on my
own waves, currents.
I'm dreaming that
I own the ocean,
the sky in total.
And can sail around
and around
without fear.
No fear of being
overtaken
by anyone or anything.
Sometimes.

Every damn day this
long list of items spreading
across the rippling field of your
mind's tired eyes. Ideations—
call them a recap, a rundown
of all wandering
accidents you've wasted
time and rumored brain
cells on. Affection, reverence,
puzzlement, disgust—one
wild and unchaperoned
barn dance you alone can
see and hear.
Older than time itself,
forever bent on renewal.

And Maybe Then

Whenever it is
that worms learn to
whistle, that's when
I'll sit down beside you
and solve the mighty lion's
share of your problems,
honey child. So try being
patient, relax, whistle
something. And maybe
then, the worms
will follow suit.

When, when
will straight flat sense
come back into use
and fashion?
Straight flat sense, in the
forthright style
favored by our moms
in the first week
of toilet training. Of course,
that's just one
example.

But wasn't Mommy
at her most loving
and pure in those days
of security and trust?
Uncluttered
and direct, like this
poem. Oh,

people today grow up
very fast, they do. Minds
corrupted so early, and usually
no undoing
the damage short of counter-
brainwashing that
promotes truth
decay. I'm dying to

get back, I'd kill to get back to
straight flat sense. What
about you?

DENNIS RIVARD

If you think
life's brutal
now...try living
about nine hundred years ago.

For every action, there's
a premonition. I have to think
so. For every
reaction, an action.
Just don't try walking backwards.

The past is pregnant
with warnings.

The future already knows
all it needs to know.
If we could only learn more
about days past,
we wouldn't worry so much
about days to come.
But, if we weren't so

worried about the future—

and what it has on us—

we'd feel emboldened to do just

as we please.

Life Coaches

Thirty years of working so
very hard, so as to get my act
into the humble column of
humility. The tidy corridor
of self-effacement, you see.
And now wouldn't you
know it? These prancing life
coaches all faulting
me for standing right
beside myself, every moment
of every little day.
Like one of those fussy
assistants in a duel.

I wonder, is this where

I go when I'm

walking in circles?

Maybe just a whacked out

question. Or maybe,

on an awfully

good day, a philosophical

question. When I don't

go inside a church is when

I feel the most

precious in God's sight.

When a spiritual

question knocks me down,

I bleed my blackest.

Here come the brightly colored
forces of evil, of dark dreams.
They are not to be
taken at face value.
I'm not sure whether they're
great at disguising or
that we by nature are born
by the minute to be fooled. Clowns
wearing tiny, metallic earpieces
line the parade route. "Security,"
it says on their funny dunce
caps. One of them has been whispering
into his plaid collar
and scowling every other minute
under his painted-on smile.
Isn't it curious that every day
one of these parades is staged
the sun comes out?
The sun is shining fiercely.
Fierce smiles line the parade route.

She says to me I don't smile
anymore. I don't
laugh. And she hints that
I need to explain. I tell her
that I wish I could.
She frowns, her frown that is
the same as mine. And I begin
to feel something like some
feathers, like feathers are
rising from a nest somewhere
inside me. But it is really
my smile. So it is.

Heads are ovals. Now it seems

my head's a race track—taken

over by fast cars and demon drivers

going nowhere ridiculously

fast and detached from

the spirit of mercy.

I found a message stuck

to my forehead: "You can keep

your little putt-putt brain,

but your mind is ours now!"

The constant roar. The eternal,

infernal blurring of every

emerging thought.

What was the start time of this?

Where is the sudden-death finish line

hidden? Pit crews with hoses

at the ready are bursting

into flames themselves.

If I pray for rain, might it rain

hard enough to turn

this track of bedlam

into one great muddy field? Because

I think the time has come

to re-define all this. Let's call it

a demolition derby.

In my glove compartment, a bottle
of artificial tears—
tossed there by me I don't
remember when. It's like a nuthouse
in there. Or a drunk tank.
White-out and crazy-glue long dried up,
useless. Plastic forks and spoons
hidden under registration,
title, proof of insurance. Alcohol
wipes. Two non-identical
tire pressure gauges—one of which
I vaguely remember
using once or twice. A few small bottles
of highly alcoholic stuff to
wash your hands with. A roll of
gauze. Stamps, envelopes, toothpaste,
toothbrush. Pair of scissors. Roll
of electrical tape. Why no
ball of string in here? You'd think...
Well, at least there's this
spool of thread, possibly in lieu of
string. Or rope. No, there'd be
no room in there for rope. An old comb—

a few teeth missing. Several

scraps of paper—on one of which this

scrawled note: "Dear God, whom we don't

understand at all, Who ARE we,

and why are we here, in this dark place?"

There Really Isn't So Much

There really isn't much left
in this so-called world of ours
that bears watching.
Let alone bear fruit.
And that's not all. I really do
find myself these days
floundering as well
as apologizing to strangers.
I think and worry way
too much about the future.
The future and the devil
may not even
exist without me projecting them
onto some inner screen.
Am I stupid to think so little
and yet so much
about the so-called future?
I mean, how much does the future
think about me?
Or even so much
as know I exist.

All my life,

I've been afraid

of being known

too well. Afraid of being

seen too clearly by the wrong

breed of snake. I

tried to project something like

those scents

that come only

from flowers. As if butterflies

would pile up in

the air wherever I

planted myself.

To protect me unwittingly.

And through a kind of

confusion,

want me.

From My Knees

Some days I feel like
Jimmy Stewart, shambling
through It's A Wonderful Life on the
power of Donna Reed's love, on
faith in the common decency
of plain people. Faith, too, in something
greater and above us.
Some days feel like traps, like low blows
waiting to be delivered
by Mr. Potter, when the money's
misplaced by the sweet, well-meaning,
absent-minded uncle.
Some days end with my worries
washed clean away by the love
of my own Donna Reed. I can rise
from my knees
and see the love of the common people
doing its simple work
in my life.

Sometimes even a fancy key
won't open a sticky door or a
tricky door. A perfect, fool-proof
key is a key bound to meet
its Waterloo. One day or another, it will
meet its match. Ironic as that
sounds. When it comes
to doors that are tricky or sticky,
sometimes force is really
the only way. Like it or not,
a heavy shoulder, a great big bloody
hammer is your best and only
bet. This isn't fascism. One day,
you'll have to find out what's
behind a certain door. Like it
or not. With some perspective—take
a few steps backward of it.
The necessity of force
in certain situations. With certain
tricky doors that stick.
Just a few steps back backward.
Perspective is the key.

They'd Be Sure To Know

If wishes were horses,
I tell you what.
I'd need to clear off hundreds
of miles to make space for
them all to graze. Feed
them top quality oats coated
with molasses and furnish
them with work they'd
naturally understand. Reasons
for waking up early,
and reasons to be tired
at the end of each long day.
In that way,
they'd be sure to know they
were horses, not just
wishes.

Always hoped and actually

thought I'd grow up

to be a fly on the wall,

some kind of poet.

Fly in the

ointment. Thought I

might just bring that ointment

down. Well,

I suppose all of that

ended up happening,

in some small way,

at least. But now

that I'm kind of turning

into an old man,

I get scared. I'm often worried

about where

the flyswatter is.

How do you and I make love?
Like the poor porcupines
in the old joke—carefully.
Old complexes, traumas and
misunderstandings are our quills.
Making love, but plenty
of other prickly situations.
Old war zones, hidden mines
that explode and big surprise booby
traps practically everywhere
we step. Or might be thinking about
stepping. These kinds
of quills are in there deeper
than anything a porcupine or
hedgehog ever dreamed of. And no
half of a quill will stick out,
waiting to be pulled out gently
by some expert
on wildlife. You'll never see
an access point for starting the rescue
operation. And any path
that ever pierced the dense forest
will have been shut down.

No notation on the map you may
have been counting on.

To Inspiration

You've got to hand it to
inspiration. Bless
its so simple heart! So
complicatedly simple a
heart! Quite smoothly,
it will return to you
all the vital
doubts and confusion that
logic had previously
pried out in
such a cool manner.

Now that Uncle Freddy's for all

intents nothing

but a big fat slob with

furtive eyes for his young

nieces and his nephew,

he's had to double

the weight of his cheesy, queasy

attempts to appear innocent vis-a-vis

the sweet, soft appeal

of quite young

flesh not yet taken. And yet, and

yet, isn't

Uncle Freddy that gentle

giant, that great shambling

bear of a man

he sees himself as

in mirrors, although not

quite so

in his own mind?

Rain

In the pouring rain, in the heavy
rainstorm, you won't be able
to engage in much of any
thinking your problems through.
But light rain's heavy mist
is the place and the time
for walking through any questions
you might have standing in your way.
For the purpose of becoming a little bit
more centered and
a little bit more circumspect,
you might add up in your head the
number of hard downpours
you've walked through
to get yourself so completely
lost in your own
small town of a life.

Our little world

is old, old. Old as hell.

One would have to be stupid

to live here and not know

it isn't young. But I theorize Life

on Earth is likely all but

neonatal. This black

ice you see everywhere—it may

well have been white

once. Our presence here—

who knows? It could have been

a very old curse. But

was it a curse on us living things,

skipping so innocently,

as we do, in ever darkening "gyres"?

Down here

in these grooves that never

go straight? Or was it

this world that ran afoul. Might we

have been sent by

"authorities" as punishment?

To punish us? Or the little old world

of ice turned black?

Quieter

Why is it never quiet?
Be quiet please, please
be still. Learn how, if you don't
know how
to be quiet. This goes
for everyone.
Everyone on the streets
and everyone else who
doesn't remember
silence. Doesn't remember,
or forgot that they ever
even knew. Ever knew
silence and how to listen
to silence till it turns
into a quiet and invisible
substance and people
can hear themselves
think and people can
remember.

The battle between a man
and his invisible enemy, depression,
is not a battle that involves
guns. Or any Medals of Honor
or otherwise. It does not call
for the spilling of any
blood, unless you spill your own,
trying to send out some sort
of distress call. A big dramatic
message you're too messed up or
too inarticulate to put
down in words. The hardest
job in the war on depression
is separating all the enemies
of your happiness and well-being
from yourself. That—as well
as the invisibility of the
whole crumby deal you deal with.
The general public doesn't
hear any sirens blaring.
No smoke burns
their eyes as you pass among them all.

Forget what maybe you've been
hearing since forever.
Love is no parasite. It isn't.
It doesn't practice sneaking
around, collecting evidence for
use against anybody.
No connection either to
rivalries, big or small. And love
has never been known much
to sulk or dissemble.
Never sinks to dredge up
suspicious evidence for use
in questionable courts.
And I'm sorry to tell you,
but love's no mythical
Greek god or goddess. Nor
any connection to the legendary
Santa Claus. No
myth, no fable. Mark my words.
Love is nothing, if not real.

Nor should you ask

that Jesus take

from you

the reins of your life.

Instead, go out looking

for a horse. One honest,

faithful

horse. And

when you

find that horse,

ride it.

When my brain has been
spilled out across the
rock-hard examination table,
all the evidence will indicate
that I was clearly
neither completely out to lunch
nor sound as a dollar. Just
like Buddha used to
say: "Hit the
ball straight back
through the middle of the field
and often it will
find its way into center
for a base hit."

He had already mastered
the game. It figured that someone
would invent it. Doubleday
or whoever—does it matter?
And the Buddha continued giving
the batter good advice, saying:
"Never take your eyes off
the outfielder. If he should appear

slack or inattentive

as he fields the ball you've hit

back through the middle,

make him pay for

letting his mind

become lazy. Take

the extra base."

Here's The Deal

Logic in action

has all the necessary moves

to bail out you and your

boat of doubt

and confusion. And by

the same token, inspiration—

with its heart full

of equal parts complication

and simplicity—

will quite happily put

the doubt and

confusion back as

a complimentary gift.

I can't recite

the alphabet anymore

in the correct order.

No more. Inside my

brain, there's a whistling

kettle. I can't turn

down the flame.

When the water's through

evaporating,

the kettle will stop

whistling, then on will

come the smoke

alarm. When the house

burns down,

there won't be any

correct order

anymore. Any alphabet

left over will

have pieces burned

off it.

Early evening shadows shadow

the late Autumn dusk. Hurtling ahead

up highway 10, feeling lost.

Ridiculous yes, but truer

than true. Heading up

to Hanover to the dentist, in

haste. Nothing familiar

anywhere along either side

of the road. Which is

scary, since I've been

up this road a thousand times

and I live only about

13 miles south.

Probably not going

to get there on time. Halloween,

and pretty fast getting

darker and darker. Dark woods

to the left and the right. With

my dementia gaining

ground. And fast. Can't even

think of the name of

this river that everyone living

anywhere near these

parts hears at least
5 times a day. Arrows on
signs everywhere I look, but
pointing to what, where?
Broken pumpkins, I've lost
count of them all.

Ocean Of Kindness

I need you, need you
so much. So much more
than you need me. Now,
or ever. You though,
you say No, it's not
like that—it's equal
and balanced, what we share
together. And equal
is constantly equal. But,
I say you only think
that it is so because you
are an ocean, an ocean
of kindness. Or else
some blind, blind river.

Even though I don't know

how to pray,

I sometimes try, but never do

get the feeling of being

pulled along into the mystic

process by

a helpful, understanding

deity. It seems both

wrong and right, the Higher

Power not reaching out a hand.

It's open to interpretation—

The silent oar, the silent lake.

The billion mile

stare. My so very frivolous

life behind

this pane of sound-proof glass.

Sound-proof glass. But is it

shatter-proof as well?

    May this question, like a cloud

        of rain, follow me

and tumble down with me,

into prayer.

A Spiritual Instinct

They could be talking

about some spiritual hint or

spiritual instinct.

But when

somebody or other

tells you they've seen

something or other,

let's say God,

in their heart,

any heart surgeon

could tell you there never

could have been any such

phenomenon.

And that

it must have

been in their

brain they saw it. But

then again, any brain

surgeon would

tell you something else.

Jaded

People have walked through
mirrors. It's been written up in
Popular Mechanics.
One time a corn dog at the Delaware
State Fair underwent
a public metamorphosis
and emerged as an ancient Greek
philosopher. He received
a big round of applause, but when
it sunk in that he couldn't
or wouldn't speak English, an angry mob
pelted him with stones and
candied apples. It truly is a shame
how Americans are
saturated with miracles.
Jaded, spoiled rotten, we insist
our miracles come smothered
in onions. On time, too,
and on demand. New episodes only.
Reruns? I don't think so.

Previously appeared in *Cape Cod Poetry Review*,
Summer 2018

DENNIS RIVARD |

The way the breezes bend young
trees is close to the way
the gentlemen once bent ladies
across the ballroom floor

while I watched through a window
at age thirteen.
This was out at the amusement park
in North Dartmouth, nearly

into Westport. Why was I there?
This was in winter—all the rides were
frozen and locked down. Why
was I there?

Oh, right—there was that dingy old
bowling alley sort of
attached to one side of the ballroom.
Went there with Audette

and Bastoni a few times. We were
teaching ourselves to bowl. Duck pins.
And it was important to put just
enough spin on the ball

to make it bend, hitting the front
pin at the perfect angle. You could
get a strike that way. Otherwise, you might
be staring at a split. Bad news.

Faint Echoes

Now I find out
I've been walking in circles
for hours, days,
years. And into the bargain,
they tell me that Ted's Variety
no longer exists. Not on the corner
of Florence and Court—
or any other corner. Now it's
no more than the faintest echo
of what I must stop
referring to as this morning.

Giving myself just
a little mid-morning
break. Even feeling
like I actually
deserve it. Looking
out through
the segmented hallway
window. See
how the sun, in its
businesslike,
"don't get
in my way" way, uses
the poor old elm
tree's sagging
arms to throw shadows
across the rest of it.

Stolen glimpses—

of human beings caught

dead or dying

on television.

We hate to hold our eyes on

them long enough

for our minds

to form memories, form

memories

that might permanently

haunt

and disable us.

0, here sit some of us

inside adequately

supplied houses. 0,

the secret life of lies.

Toying with ideas

about the secret

life of God. 0, the dirty

life of flies.

Money is his mother,

power is his father.

And when he

prays to them—on

rare occasions—

they fall down laughing.

And never incur

injury.

The Martians

You could go fishing.

I've heard this place is

the water planet.

The Martians call it that,

according to reports.

They have perspective

and see us for

what we really are: fish

out of water.

I admire the Martians.

They do not covet

all these lakes and oceans.

Nor cool streams and rushing

rivers. I'm sure they could use some

cool water. It is truly

a planet on fire, Mars

is, and we named it

after some fictional god

of war. Yet they are all about

peace and dignity,

despite the ferocity of red heat

they constantly

have to deal with. They can't

go fishing, but they do
not covet. You've got to
admire that.

Or July In New Hampshire. I ask
myself:
What if these roadblocks turn out
to be safety nets? What if
pushing my way through
them proves to be nothing
but the first stop
of my approach to further roadblocks?
More subtle yet harsher.
What if my future holds
nothing more of the gentle than
a coma? What if
the highest highlight of future life
proves to be on a par with this
watching that I'm doing right
this moment? This watching, that is,
of a hefty woman
and her just as hefty man as they
do their approach
to Ramunto's Pizza? Slowly drifting
across this parking lot
on foot, melting
tar underneath their feet?

I'd have thought
you'd have made some kind
of contact by now.
Phone call, text message,
something. Easily
enough done. Just a matter
of wanting to extend
a hand, virtual or otherwise.
I could see it if we were living
in the world of a hundred
years ago, when the wheels all
turned much slower. That is,
if they turned at all.
And here I am, talking
to myself again.

It's always a good thing
to go around angry
for 5 or 6 days minus
knowledge of why.
That's how poems and sometimes
babies are conceived. That's
correct, the darkness. Right—
the passionate power of opposing forces
in the dark. Covers thrown off,
pulled back, and thrown off again.
The moon's silent hands
doing God knows
what to the tides.

The suitability of the container

and the power of the darkness

to deceive. The gift

of life was a heavy gift.

Heavier than he had

ever suspected. He thought the

second-hand gym bag

from the nearby thrift store

would be strong enough

for holding it,

transporting it.

He figured

the distance

wrong too. The container,

the weight, the power. He was

overwhelmed

and deceived in darkness.

Reporting From Depression

Crows don't represent anything,

and a freezing, stubbled

cornfield in January

means nothing. A gray squirrel

runs from my yard

and doesn't stop until it knows

it's safe from me, up

in Laurie's dying poplar tree.

There's a hard edge on every surface.

The sun withdraws its rays

and puts on a pained expression.

A small plane disappears

behind a cloud

on its way to nowhere.

Nowhere, the most popular destination.

Even though I don't know

how to pray, I try hard

to figure it out

on my own. Without having

to go out and get some

manual or other.

I always fall into the false

hope that if I go to all

the trouble of sitting still

for however many minutes,

leaving myself

open to the whims

of the idiots who jabber

always inside my

head, God will

cut me some slack and

chime in.

Sink Or Swim

The fact is
that we climbed up
from the mud and slime
at the farthest depths
and have been trying to live here
in this new and different world.
A better world in most
respects, though we had hope
of leaving mud and slime
behind. It sounds simple
as I report it now,
but it wasn't. We had that
eons-long layover
as creatures of the sea. To say
the least, it's been a very slow transition.
Sink or swim—that's been
the deal all along.
On the ocean floor, you could crawl
in darkness forever. Forever,
or until eaten by some blind,
unidentified thing.
That kind of history doesn't get
erased overnight.

Blackberry Hill, Black Cloud

Tall fences
keep me from knowing
my good neighbors. I trust
these virtual strangers
to behave according
to their reputations, even as I
build a bonfire
for the flaming execution of all
things past. Meanwhile, my mind
is telling me what my heart
can't—that those crushing and tearing
sounds being
carried up the hill
by the nagging winds of late February
aren't any reinforcement
brigade.

All of the above are

accidents you have wasted

your life and time

with. And there aren't

any reasons that hold

water for you

having done it.

No apparent reasons,

no. But

just as poems might

sink or float

on what would appear

to be just

driftwood, this life

goes and comes

according to

the needs of absentee

acrobats and unseen

ballet masters.

The thing about sharks is

that they never stop moving.

But it doesn't seem

to be causing them

to lose much sleep.

I've never seen one

looking sleepy and

haggard.

I know it wasn't

a curse cast over them, like

with the

Gypsies, who haven't

been able to stop rambling

for a couple of thousand

years now.

I guess it's just

a metastatic

experience. A life-long romance

with the joy of movement.

Adrenaline's good

when you need to lift

a Toyota Corolla

off your 6 year old child

in a hurry. And

if you're working

behind a convenience

store counter, a loud-talking,

big-bellied, old

blowhard prone to flashing

some phoney

special deputy badge

every time he opens

his wallet to pay

for scratch-off tickets

will never do you any favors.

Also, I've learned

not to trust

my own judgment

when precision

instruments are easily

obtainable in certain

stores and catalogs, but

by the same token,

there are a few things

unmeasurable by anything

besides one's own

gut feeling.

Something's wrong, something's wrong—
when you can't go out
for a quart of milk
without dying inside
a ten-gallon hatful of
World Friction. Once upon
a time, this country
consisted of mainly
cattlemen. Cattlemen, farmers, and
more farmers. Then the sheep
were brought over.
And it was all but over after that.

And if I sing of the joys
of patience. And if I
lock myself down in the chamber
of bottomless patience.
And if I hang tough, enveloped
in some righteous cloud or
other, for inspiration—
sweet inspiration—to drift
through my doorway and pop
a few wheelies on
the gangplank of my imagination.
For crying out loud, I'll
be asleep and dreaming by the
time she makes it
here to me. And, God knows,
it might prove out to be not
She herself, but rather
just some opportunistic and
ambitious flunkie. I mean,
just some out of work
part-timer off the street.
I refuse to embarrass
myself so.

Rhode Island

I can't balance a checkbook
or figure out how many
miles I'm getting per gallon.
I struggle to find my way
out of Concord, New Hampshire.
Really can't recite a passage
from Shakespeare any longer than
ten words. To be or not to be—
that's kind of an offbeat question.
And yet, I ask it every day. In one
way or another. Who doesn't?
My auto technician, that's who?
It's because he's mechanically inclined
and has accepted Jesus as
his personal savior. He can balance
his checkbook, too. Not Jesus,
but Jamie. But I myself have trouble
not getting lost in Providence,
Rhode Island. The road signs
are few, and they don't make a whole
lot of sense. At least not to me.
In fact, all of Rhode Island
is very mysterious—if not outright

nightmarish. It's impossible
to get out of it, if you don't know
what you're doing, think the world is
out to get you, and feel like
there's nothing deep inside that you
might fashion into a tool. More specifically,
a dangerous weapon.

I'm not the least bit happy
with you and your obsessions
creeping over here, so close to my
own. Here on my own little
beach blanket I'd rather sprawl
here by myself, absorbing
the sounds of the sun and the rays
of the blazing ocean. Your
little obsessions are far too naked
to be dancing here in my
private space. I mean, have they
no shame? Like you must
have raised them up on the topless
beaches of Brazil. And
they'd be rudely blocking out
the plangent music
of the sun in the sky if it weren't so
directly above, at 12 o'clock. Those
are not the obsessions
I used to think could blend
comfortably with mine.
Saw myself as watching them swim
in your womb, alongside my

own obsessions. Until the time
came to be reborn. In my crazed
imagination, they were swelling, swelling.
Like tides in your deep, dark fathoms.

Sudden And Abrupt

I want to push the world

down a whole flight of stairs.

Wheelchair and all, I swear.

Just like Richard Widmark,

in The Kiss Of Death. Brutal.

Sudden and abrupt, in black

and white. Call it

revenge, catharsis, or vigilante

justice. Whatever.

I've got a million reasons and the laugh

of a maniac. I owe no one

any explanation.

When does a whim start

calling itself

a heavenly

impulse?

When is it that

death

starts being

introduced as

an inspired

culmination?

A clicking inside

my head

has been a pain

in the ass to me

for it seems

like a hundred years.

I swear I'm

soon going to start calling it

some kind of

epiphany.

Here, we are, Mom, on the

senile dementia side of life.

Just kidding. Here we are, though

on the senile dementia side

of Sacred Heart nursing home

and rehab. No, you don't have to

be Catholic. It's OK, they take

everyone here. It's where you

live now. Janet and Nancy

and I come and visit you

when we can get here. Church

people sometimes, too.

That guy you thought was your

insurance man yesterday? You'll

think this is pretty funny—

that was Reverend Peters, the new

minister at St. Paul's.

Listen to that, Mom...somebody's

having a birthday party

across the hall. No, not for you, for

the man across the hall. I wish

you had a better view out your window.

The Acushnet River runs

right behind that old warehouse.

Don't cry—it's just that guy's family

singing Happy Birthday. No,

don't cry. It isn't scary music. It's not

scary music at all, Ma.

Vanity And Ego

Well enough fed,
but not feeling it.
Sitting on a fortune in
gold, but delaying
it. Oh mercy!
Vanity and ego, the usual
suspects, coming for
me again. Shouldn't they
respect me at least
an ounce? An iota?
Who do they think's been
supporting them,
all these years?

Worn down to the nub
by your spirit—by your
nothin' doin', new
personality and spirit—

I go outside and walk a bit.
And come back—
thinking, when
you ask me where did I

go, I'll say nowhere. Just
went out to look
for a new pencil.

Assertive, uninhibited, never
out of control. That's what
she tells me I should be.
These therapists seem to think
I should be—and can be—some kind
of miracle man.
So here I am, driving
home, crossing over
the deep, dark
Connecticut River. Getting dark
out here. Bits and pieces
of not quite snow, not quite cold, stinging
rain, attacking my
windshield.
A slippery bridge? I hope not.
God I hope not.

On To The Next Phase

When it was staying
here with us, in our
house, it lived in a kitchen
cupboard. That was when it was a can of
Progresso vegetable soup.
Where it went from here,
whatever new form
it took, your guess is
as good as mine.

Somewhere Out Of Reach

There was a day that went by,
barely registering, some
years back. It was the day
you fell into the habit
of keeping your doors
and windows
locked at all times. Even
the doors of your car,
while driving it six blocks
to the Laundromat.
At your house—although it isn't
something you're completely
conscious of—you're afraid
someone will somehow get in
through an opening not
nailed shut. Even when seated
at the living room window,
considering a warm, red
sunset. There's no
way to track that day down
and erase its every whisper
from the history of your thoughts.
It's gone now, it's nowhere.

Somewhere

where you can't get at it.

Reality has picked up a habit
of turning into total
confusion, or something.
She used to be someone you could
set your bedside clock to.
But now, I don't understand her
habits. She's getting old, perhaps,
I guess. But then again it just isn't easy
to believe she was ever really
young. But she used to
do calisthenics and balance her and
other people's checkbooks
with an incredible precision, just
for fun.
She used to be the essence
of kindness, yes—
but also of rational thinking
and action. Ah, but
now...now she calls me
by the wrong name. She leaves
her hat on in the house.
She reels when standing up from
her old stuffed chair. Twice,

she asked me if I still

could walk on my hands. As if

I ever could.

Reality is going senile; the world is

showing wear and hard use.

Rivers and meadows

and tall trees, they seem

to know their way around.

Appear to know their purpose

in life, if I'm not stretching

to presume too much. And mountains

can be brutal, might terrorize.

But never not for

no reason. You just need to

know the facts.

And then, there's gravity.

In the final analysis, gravity

holds sway over all of it.

And what right have we

to complain or deny?

We've been here a much shorter

time.

A thousand questionable

reasons to stay home

kicking myself

and treating the bruises

with kisses. Just one

reason—questionable at

best—to step out

into the streets. Onto the streets

that people of sound

minds know

are dangerous,

narrow

passages through stolen

mountains. The explosions

will echo through the streets

forever or until old,

devouring gods return

to re-take them.

She always did
want to be some sort
of big-shot. And wouldn't
you know it, there she sits
meditating. Her followers
are right there, in a circle around
her. Nothing between
her bottom and the hardwood
floor but one thin
prayer mat. She's got a bunch
of books about the spirit
and the light
within out there on the
Spirituality market, so I've heard.
I may be the only one
here who knows her name
used to be Elizabeth.
But who cares? Most people
contemplate name changes
and some go through
with it. It's a secret dream of
many others. One thing
I know—she

won't stop until she's up
among the stars and all
the top gurus.

It's no longer possible to be
born in a fresh, clean world.
Pre-owned is all that's left. Don't
take it personally. Sure, it's less
than pleasant and delightful
when some mangy old fox—sick
as a dog—staggers out of
the woods and slowly gives up
the ghost in your own
back yard. Right beside the jungle
gym, too. Grotesque?
Sure it is. But still, Vermont's a far
cry from a Third World country, where
it could easily have been
your grandmother crawling out of
those woods to die as
close to you as possible.
You might say this incident
with the mangy old fox
was, relatively
speaking, a kind of blessing.

There must be something I can do.
I've got a deck of 52 cards
that keeps on
shuffling in my heart.

And another deck, missing
3 cards, is rumored to be
lost in my head.
Perhaps not

coincidentally, 3 lost cards
are rumored to be stuck

in my throat, having
shimmied up the greased pole
of my heart.

On the top floor
of the towering building,
the features that beleaguer me sit
on their fat asses. Yes, Mr. Self-Doubt
and Mr. Self-Pity, entrenched
in their corner offices.
They've got the ways and means—
and the perfect vantage point—
to see all challengers
coming, and to
repel them. Challengers are for pushing
out the windows of the soul, so that
they plummet with legs and arms
flailing and end up
nothing more, nothing more
than additional smudges
on the hard pavement.

Now I'm shut off and shut out.

Mr. Self-Doubt and Mr. Self-Pity.
I remember how they seemed,
years and years ago, when

they first showed up here—

calling themselves Humility and

Tolerance. They seemed

so gentle and so necessary. And so,

I hired them to run this

business I'd inherited—so small

and fragile then. Hired them without

a second thought.

A poem can be a heavy
load of mail, borne by
a thin pony. Express, across
the happy hunting grounds
of the lonely planet.

    As it nears the station,
it has no intention

    of stopping. It looks
like some blind pony, a pony that
has lost its mind.

    But on and on
it goes,
chasing down a scent, a wild
scent—in
the spirit of the eternal
letter not sent.

You're always hearing

the totally strange scientific

fact that caterpillars

somehow manage

to change into butterflies.

You hear it pretty often.

And why the Hell

not, I guess. Okay,

I'm starting to

believe it. I suppose

if they're careful

about what they eat and are

kind and considerate

to strangers

and the vulnerable.

I know that with faith,

perhaps,

anything's possible.

For butterflies, for anyone.

The Face Of The Earth

I'm a lusting, needful creature
and I stumble along in step
with the pack. We get
in each other's ways more
or less routinely. How could
we not? Covering the face
of Earth, as we must, criss-crossing
into either ugly or
beautiful mix-ups not to be
examined. Never mind understood.
No vacation time, no
holidays worth mentioning.
Loving and hurting, hating and
forgetting to wonder. Go ahead,
label them consequences,
but in fact they are
hobbies.

It's not your imagination.
My eyes have been removed
and replaced by two shiny
buttons. Now I'm no
longer bothered by glare or
those troublesome shadows
that were the cause of my walking
into things, into places
we're not allowed to visit. Not
even for a moment. Free of charge,
those government people
put me to sleep, got rid
of my eyes that had gone bad
anyway, and woke me
up again. Now I can see
what I was missing out on: brilliant
colors that don't fatigue
the buttons of my eyes or mind.
Colors that are bold and
delightful, without arousing any
nasty fears or ideas.

Yesterday I felt like Big Chief Broom,

the silent giant in "One Flew Over

The Cuckoo's Nest." I was

immobilized

by a fear so heavy and immense that

words to describe it

haven't yet visited our planet. But still,

no one dared look me

in the eye, and I possessed some small

measure of control.

Today, on the other hand, I feel

like Gulley Jimson—hero of

"The Horse's Mouth." I'm fueled by

a boundless reservoir

of nerve and crazed bravado, pissing off

people everywhere with my

driving. I refuse to recognize the center

line of any road I take to. I am

utterly surrounded, this very

moment, by a thousand

beautiful butterflies.

On waking up from
another sterilized hospital
dream, I smell it, I
spot it inside the wide open
little bedside table
drawer. Don't think it
was me who left it open.
But a white styrofoam cup
of black coffee sits in there.
A strange place for it to be,
but so it is. Healthcare
being sometimes hard to recognize.
My assumption, just about,
would be it was put there by
that jive talking speech
therapist. The coffee looks
embarrassed, at that, to be
in there. If it had ears,
I'd tell it I feel
out of place here myself.

Curling Iron

Wiped out on so
many levels, I couldn't
begin to tell you.
So many of my mind's branches
closed because they couldn't
be salvaged. Now, just
a lucky few branches
still up and running—on double
and triple shifts. And whatever
hard tasks and philosophical
questions might come to litter
the in-box will be
put to a hard test to prove
they merit my attention
in the slightest. And time is
running down like
an old junk curling iron.

I broke your fall,

when you were falling

into a place I saw

as dangerous, if not

downright evil.

And if it was more like

a case of something

more good than bad,

I didn't know how to look

at it that way.

Imagined, maybe, that voice

that called for me to

take action. And into that

shadowy something, I

broke your fall.

You can learn to read lips
or read tea leaves.
You can learn to read palms
or autopsy reports.
Do you prefer to look at paintings
that release you into the winds of
abstraction, allow
thoughts and feelings to wander?
Or do you dream of piloting
fighter jets—working with instruments
and signals to execute
a mission crisply?

You think you see where this
is headed. You think
you see which side I'm coming from.

I don't care. I admire
the sight of how a sound
will scatter the crows in an instant.
A telephone wire abandoned.
I'm impressed and always
amazed to see a fighter jet

land so precisely on a postage stamp

deck space and stick there.

The Swinging

Another nice case
of betwixt and between.
It seems to suit me.
Creamy pink
and egg yolk yellow-orange
sunrise in full-slow swing,
across the horizon.
And it enters my mind that
on the other side
of the world so enigmatic,
it's sundown. It's
a conclusion. And for crying
out loud, here's me. In
quiet and mostly fair
Vermont, not wanting to
get in the way of
such a case of friction.
A window sitter, a fixture.

They ought to call this pathway
Confusion Boulevard,
maybe. But no—being so
forgetful and confused is more like
walking around in an alleyway
that gets longer and shorter
and goes from much too wide
to pressing way hard
in on you. And then, you won't
recall how you even
got there or why.
And you might not even
dare to ask. People around you
get so sick of you asking.

As we spend our time
on this Planet Earth, it might
be an essential necessity
that we take the time
to look at the flora, the fauna,
the actions moving over
and under and through...

That we take the time to follow our wonder.
And,
not to pretend that ugliness
and hatred and fear
aren't spread around
like rats amid mountains
of teeming waste...

That we take the wonder and the
beauty of the natural world—what's left—
as intense instruction
toward the love and truth...

of God. Our souls,
our blood, our backyard trees.

When inspiration
steps up upon
your unkempt,
forlorn
doorstep,

you probably should go
to the door, open it
with a laid-back smile.
Be nice to it,

thank it for coming.
And without
sounding greedy,

say something like
"It's been awhile, good
to see you again.

So—what have you got
today
for me?"

Walking through K-Mart,
like the lab rat you can feel
yourself becoming. Through K-Mart,
along strangely staggered aisles
that are piping out Christmas tunes
that likely have been
altered to allow for
the subliminal messages
K-Mart surely must have a
hand in. Staggered aisles that are
encouraging you somehow to
find more money in your heart so
you can visit the aisles
you've never paid any attention to.
Like some lab rat, with weighted K-Mart
shoes on. Weighted for God knows
what purposes.
The weighted shoes
on your tiny, mutated feet.
The lab rat you feel
yourself becoming.

There's a cloud skimming across
the sky above my head, looking
like a huge battleship, no end to
its whiteness. And I,
sitting miles below, can only make
an uneducated guess at
its size, its ghostly dimensions.
All I have between
myself and the green stretch
of springtime grass is a plastic
and rubber contraption shaped to
resemble an electric chair. Minus
the electricity—thank you kindly.
And I can only imagine how much
trouble this easygoing town
would be facing, were
this battleship above my head
not just a single cloud.
Only a drifter.

I know a good many people
for whom life is more
sprint than marathon.
They would tell you that cheating
is fine and OK,
if you're fast enough
to make it secret from the judges.
And the media.

And the judges overseeing
these sporting events, these
races, well... they've been
around the block a time or two.
And so they say
to the sprinters, Feel free.
Do what you gotta do. The
fines we don't collect from you,

We make up for on the marathoners.
An honest and methodical bunch
they are, suckers for
punishment to begin with.
Time will tell.

If only it were that

simple, I keep

on thinking. To just go back

and make a few small

changes. Simple. The poem of

one's life. Make a tweak

here or there. A different

rhythm, different word.

Lock in the changes

and pray not

to have miscalculated.

If only it were.

When the black-clad man

says go on and choose

your weapons,

you—predictably—pick

that heavy, bejeweled sword

that glitters, but only

when the sun favors it

with a glance. That

sword is called "The letter

of the law." The other

man in the duel

likes to dance and sing; he selects

the lighter, more flexible

sword. That sword is

whip-thin and it twirls

like a ballerina in the air.

Its name, of course, is "Spirit,"

and it is bound to cut

you down to size

in any fair fight.

Can't help but think

that poets have something

like a duty I guess

to try

bringing some cheer to the low

in spirit.

One way

or another, and also

a responsibility

to bring some gloom

up close

to those who would otherwise be

missing out on the pearls

of wisdom

that come along attached

to the very bottom

of depression's most impressive

boat. And you could call it

a lifeboat, maybe. I'm not sure

I can say. But one could.

Here Are The Numbers

Hindsight is 20/20. The chances
of your holy matrimony
ending in divorce are 50/50.
Odds of you becoming a star
in Hollywood or in professional sports
are a million to one. Someone spotting the
Blessed Virgin Mary's face
on a bruised apple at their local
Price Chopper in the next week is
about a 6-to-1 shot.
Nine times out of ten, the victim
knew their assailant. Should an accident
take place, it will happen at home,
nine times out of ten.
A flipped coin is just as likely
to come up heads
a hundred straight times as it is
just once. At least in theory. In reality,
zero chance. About one-in-five
of us humans are aware of being
"queer." I'm using
about 8% of my brain's potential when
writing a poem, and about

twice that when thinking up
vain lies.

You May Not Know This

There is only one way to tell
snowstorms you're not
gonna take it anymore, lying down
or standing up. You can either
buy a shovel—aluminum
surface if you can—
or cure yourself of
dandruff with a banana
split and a little
turpentine.

I pick up the guitar
of your heart yet again
and try, one last time,

to play the song right.
You Are My Sunshine.
But it seems like

the strings have changed.
The sound doesn't
flow right. The timing

and my fingers are
so hard to coordinate.
The least complicated song

one could wish for.
My fingers have gotten away
from simplicity.

World's Strongest

Like the world's
strongest man breaking

up a barroom fight,
sunlight—weighing in at

less than what a fraction
of one feather

might weigh—
pushes all the clouds aside.